Enjoy Your Wardrobe

How to declutter and
discover your treasures

Lena Bentsen

Declutter expert and Danish Life Designer

ISBN-13: 978-1978109971
ISBN-10: 1978109970

Printed in the United States of America

Why did I write this book?

I wrote this book because I would like to help you experience the beautiful feeling of freedom that comes from having a wardrobe holding only your very best clothing and accessories – your treasures. A wardrobe with only your treasures is a step towards Danish Hygge. Since 2005 I have helped numerous families get a unique home with spirit, charm and Danish Hygge by cleaning up, organizing and decorating with care and I want to share the method with you.

Why should you read this book?

You should read this book if you are tired of opening your wardrobe every day and not knowing what to wear because there is not enough clothing that feels right. If you would like to know how to distinguish between clothing to be kept and what needs to be removed, you should read this book without delay.

What can this book help you with?

This book will help you say goodbye to clothing without having a bad conscience - and help you to enjoy the clothes you keep. It is the ultimate guide to obtaining the most personalized wardrobe you could wish for, so that in the future, you will only have to choose clothing according to mood and occasion because everything is 100% you.

What some readers have to say

"It was a great feeling to trim down my wardrobe with you by my side in the book. I have never felt so happy throwing out so many clothes." – Ulla, Copenhagen

"When I got rid of many clothes, the picture of my wardrobe changed. Suddenly I could see the hidden style and color code. Hurry to read this book." – Anne, Aarhus

About The Author

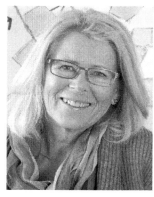 Lena Bentsen, born in 1954, is known as "The Grand Old Lady" in the Danish decluttering business. In 2005, she started the organization wave in Denmark. As a trained Feng Shui interior designer, she also knows, feels, and sees the details of a space that can provide or disrupt the feeling of wellbeing.

As a native Dane, Danish Hygge flows through her veins and is a part of her DNA. During her lifetime, Lena Bentsen has become intimately familiar with every Danish tradition. As a Danish Life Designer, she paints the picture of the deepest essence of Danish Hygge and the typical Danish way of life. To gain the feeling and spirit of Danish Hygge, it is a must to care about your home and life – and decluttering is therefore essential.

Lena Bentsen is a famous author in Denmark, who has written several books about these topics. She and her work often attract media attention.

Table of Contents

A Foreword about Danish Hygge and Clutter

Maybe you have heard that Danish people are among the happiest people in the world and that Danish hygge is something very special. It is true, but we are not born this way. It is in our culture, and it can be learned. Even you can learn it.

Hygge is difficult to describe, but the essence of hygge is a moment filled with joy, peace and harmony. A moment where nothing can hurt you. A moment with no place for worries – only the deepest feeling of, yes, joy, peace and harmony.

Here comes the big secret: To gain this spirit of hygge, you have to take care of your surroundings by decluttering, caring and focusing on the details.

Clutter is your hidden enemy. I'm definitely not advocating hysterical decluttering, but I am advocating having a home filled with your personality. A home with a beating heart. Your home.

In this book, I will help you become best friends with your wardrobe. I will help you to figure out which clothing in your wardrobe has a special place in your heart. Once you know and feel this, you will get a bit closer to the inner feeling of Danish Hygge.

A Welcome from Me to You

Dear Reader,

I sincerely want to welcome you, because I know you have bought this book with the decision to make some changes in your life.

Decluttering your wardrobe with me is not simply decluttering. When you look through your treasures hidden amongst all the things in your wardrobe, you will unveil the true version of YOURSELF. You will become unique.

Every day you are painting a picture of who you are from top to toe. The saying "Fine feathers make fine birds" also applies to you. Your clothes tell everything about who you are and who you want to be. Believe me.

This book will help you to finally overcome the challenges of the past—standing in front of your wardrobe frustrated and in despair, not knowing what to wear. The amount of clothing that you need will be personal. Only you know what kind of clothes will bring you the great feeling of freedom.

I hope that with order, you will have the best of luck finding all the good things in your life that have been hiding. I will help you through this with humour and a supportive hand. Let's get started.

Do You Recognize this Situation?

But I really don't have any clothing...! Have you ever wondered why it seems impossible to find decent clothing to wear, even though your wardrobe is overflowing?

How many times has your boyfriend or husband replied: "How can it be so difficult to find something with all the clothes you have?"

Well yes, but it's not just about clothing. There are lots of other things in a wardrobe that should help us create the best version of ourselves.

Even though everyday life can be confusing with ordinary, every-day matters, no two days are the same. We dress by occasion and because there are a lot of different occasions, it is clear to anyone with a proper wardrobe that we, of course, need different clothing. A lot of clothing.

The danger of having A LOT of clothing for MANY occasions is simply that we do not get to use them as much as we intended when we bought them.

Another pitfall could be that we really do not know our own clothing type; are we a bit bohemian, or would it be better to look like a million dollars? But none of these clothing types have lasted. Maybe you are just completely different. Maybe you are just you?

It sure can be difficult figuring out your style. There is not much else to do except try. Many people would like to help you if they were being paid. I'll pass—not for me.

A third pitfall is fashion. Fashion tends to change and who does not want to look like they are up-to-date? But that does not mean that yesterday's fashion clothing is disposable—just a small, but very important chapter, which could be named...:

It might be in fashion again!

I see incredible amounts of clothing in wardrobes where the owner, with great certainty and belief, claims that fashion changes and that clothing that was in fashion ten years ago will be in fashion again. Nothing is more wrong. Fashion never returns in the exact same version, nor will you be the same ten years from now. Believe me.

Forget everything about saving clothing hoping that the retro style will justify keeping it. If you reuse old clothing from the past, you will only look like—sorry to say—a remnant from the past. Avoid this.

Much More than Clothing

A wardrobe is not just home to clothing. A wardrobe consists of many, many different things. We will get into most of them here. Maybe you have all of them in your wardrobe, maybe some are in closets and drawers elsewhere in the house. Regardless, I believe you know where. It is even possible that you have something in your wardrobe, which I have not thought of at all.

Clothing

Underwear - socks - blouses of all kinds - shirts - sweaters - cardigans - pullovers - jackets - outerwear - work clothes - casual wear - seasonal clothes - party clothes - yard clothes - clothes for painting - dresses - tunics - ponchos - etc.

Accessories

Jewellery - watches - scarves - bags - suitcases - belts - hair accessories - clothing jewellery...

Shoes

Summer shoes - winter shoes - outdoor shoes - indoor shoes - morning shoes - evening shoes - party shoes - casual shoes - high-heeled shoes - sneakers - spectacle shoes (shoes with heels so high that it is only possible to stand and look good) - ski boots - bathing shoes - rubber boots - winter boots...

Shoe accessories - shoe bags - shoe boxes…

It is a struggle to make room for all of it. We will get into most of it in the book.

Who are You?

In order for you to start selecting the very best of your clothing, we need to set some criteria for the selection. You have to realize that some things—or many—have to be thrown out or passed on. It will not become more spacious if you just adjust the piles and put the shoes in line. Of course, you should do this, but it is absolutely last on the agenda.

When selecting clothing you want to keep, you need to understand your own values. The old saying: "Clothes make the man" is just as applicable now as it was 1000 years ago.

Whether we want to or not, we always dress according to our circumstances. If you have a meeting with the bank, you do not show up in jogging clothes. If you are going skiing, you do not bring summer clothes. If you are going to the forest, you do not wear stilettos.

We wear clothing that fits the occasion, and clothing tells a story about us that we want it to tell in a given situation. Some say they do not care at all about what clothing they wear. This is not true. Some may be less aware of what they wear than others, but not caring—not true.

If you do not know your clothing type, it can be a very good—and financially responsible—idea to figure this out. Once you know your clothing type, you will avoid countless shopping mistakes. A lot of clothing in your wardrobe could be one of these mistakes. It looked so great in the store and you would actually not mind adding a more feminine touch to your wardrobe. Unfortunately, it did not go as expected, and now that flowery thing clings to the hanger like a bad conscience every time you see it. It is still nice, but you are not going to wear it. You just do not feel like yourself in it. You do not sing the same song. You are not in harmony—or however else we could phrase it, but one thing is certain, you will never be the best couple because you do not suit each other.

When you soon begin to rip out your wardrobe, think about what story you want to tell about yourself.

Dressing is a personal matter. Therefore, only you know what clothing is you. All I ask is for you to choose the highest common denominator. Do not settle for less and keep clothes that are not you. If so, I believe it is better to do without it.

It is better to do without than settling for less

When choosing clothing you want to keep, choose the best. Whether it is for your daily work or it is the clothing you wear when painting or when you are in the garden, it should fit the occasion.

From my own world

I often go to a wonderful small island in Denmark. An island so far from the mainland that life simply has a completely different pace there. The tempo is different. The inhabitants of the island have their own calmness. You should never rush someone from this island.

And here it comes. Just because it is far away, because you will probably not bump into your neighbour or business associates there, and because you are on vacation, you do not have to show up in the local corner store looking completely ridiculous with your Hawaiian shorts, fat stomach and straw hat—with socks in your clogs.

Maybe you want to appear totally relaxed with a farewell to civilization, but you can do this at home in the garden. One must have respect for one's own self-esteem and particularly for the people you meet—also at the corner store! Every outfit in due time. Even in holiday country.

The 100%
Your Wardrobe in Total

In a fairly ordinary wardrobe without a recent clean up, we can divide the 100% into the good ol' 80/20 rule.

There are only two categories in your wardrobe. Wearing/not wearing. That's it.

1. Clothes you wear - that is the 20%
2. Clothes you do not wear - that is the 80%

As you know 80% is 4 times more than 20%. Obviously, it can be a bit difficult to find the golden 20% amongst the 100%!

There might be many reasons for clutter in your wardrobe. Your overflowing closet might not be overflowing because you have kept clothing since your youth. It might be because you just have too much in relation to your usage. Nice, useful, modern clothing, but too much of it.

The 20%
The 20% is clothing you wear. Like, really wear. Not clothing that could be worn, but isn't, because then we are dealing with the 80%. Be very aware of this difference.

There is so much we can wear,
but so little we actually wear
— and even less we need, even though it is useful!

Clothing you wear, like really wear, can be divided into 2 categories:
- Clothing you wear all the time—depending on the season
- Clothing you rarely wear—special occasions

We have our favourite clothing. Clothing that we wear all the time—almost regardless of the season. In winter, a cardigan is worn over the blouse together with a scarf, and in summer the same blouse is worn, but together with something else.

Clothing you rarely use might be nice for parties, or for occasions like a ski trip or when it is time to paint. It is still clothing you use, but rarely. Of course, it should not stop you from being critical once it is pulled out of the wardrobe.

That was the 20%. They are as such not a problem—except that they are hiding.

The 80%
The 80% is clothing you do not wear. Remember, we are talking about you. This is where you need to focus on clothing that you do not wear. The reason is completely irrelevant now. It simply concerns clothing you do not wear.

In the section for clothing you do not wear, there are only two categories as well:

1. Clothing that is useful
2. Clothing that is not useful

That's it.

For example, have you spent too much money on a piece of clothing that turned out not to be your best friend? Well, the damage is done and you will not become richer, nor more beautiful by saving the magnificent piece one year more.

Useful clothing

Useful clothing is clothing that can be worn by others, but is not worn by you. It could be:

- Outdated clothing, but still nice and pretty.
- Somewhat expensive clothing when purchased, and now you are reluctant to get rid of it.
- Clothing that does not fit anymore. We will not get into why…!
- A lot of specific clothing, which means you cannot wear it all.
- Clothing you were tempted to buy, but have never worn. In the end, it turned out not being your style.

Not useful clothing

Not useful clothing is clothing that cannot or should not be worn by others. It could be:

- Ruined clothing that you haven't repaired.

- Clothing that is no longer nice due to wear or a stubborn stain.
- Clothing that has been washed too many times—or maybe incorrectly.
- Clothing without its companion—such as socks.
- Smelly clothing.

Moving On...

Clothing, like so many other belongings in our lives, comes and goes. Though there seems to be a tendency for more to come than to go!

And here is the fourth pitfall: when we have too much clothing, we do not have a clear picture of what we have or what we need. This is a situation that can quickly lead to impulse buying here-and-there that you think you may need or believe will do wonders for your wardrobe.

A Little Preparation

Before you get started, you have to prepare. You must do a couple of purchases. Sorry, no new clothing. Not right now at least, but a few practical arrangements.

Garbage bags

Buy plenty of garbage bags of the kind you use in your municipality. And I really mean PLENTY. Not because everything is being thrown out, but because you will need them.

You will need bags for:
- Clothing to the second-hand store
- Clothing for second-hand/sale with friends
- Clothing to be thrown out

Labels

In order to mark the bags, you will need to buy fairly large stickers/labels. Once the bags are packed and closed, you immediately have to be able to see where the bag is going.

They can simply be white labels, on which you put a large coloured cross to signify where the bag is going, or write a note who the recipient is.

Forget about post-it notes. They fall off and if you put them in the bag, they will quickly disappear in the clothes.

Passing on

Bags must be passed on as quickly as possible. It is better to do one extra trip than to take the risk of the bags being stuck at home again.

Bags to be picked up must be gone
within maximum 14 days.

A small tip

To close a bag, spread the top half flat out and roll it down from the top until you reach the content. Grab the two sides of the folded section and tie a double knot. You can hold this knot with one hand and carry the bag as a handbag. You can even carry two at once. It is much better for your back to carry bags this way than just tying a knot without rolling it first—that makes a bad grip.

Storage boxes

You will also need storage boxes. Good, identical, solid, square boxes, but do not buy these boxes until you know what you need.

You will use the boxes to store seasonal clothing in. More on this later.

To recap:

- Garbage bags (plenty)
- Labels (big ones)
- Storage boxes (wait)

It is Time to Ask Some Questions

The trick is figuring out what clothing is going into what category. If it was so easy, you probably would have already cleaned out your wardrobe... My advice is: talk to your clothing. I know it sounds childish and it is going to sound a bit funny when you have a good talk with a pair of underwear, but putting it into words for you to hear, makes a difference.

Once you have gotten used to focusing on each piece of clothing separately, there is no need for a long talk every time. You will quickly know the answer, but start by being on the same wavelength with things and talk. Of course, some clothes can immediately be pulled off the shelf or hanger and put into the right bag, but you will question a lot as well.

Obviously, you have a lot in your closet that you are happy with, but that is not the same as wearing it. Or ever wearing it in the future. Maybe the time has not been right for you to be concrete and look at it with determination. It is time now!

Start talking to your clothes now, so you are sure of the answer.

"When did I wear you last?"

You might stand with the nifty little New Year's dress in your hand and obviously you only wear it on very rare occasions. But you have to be honest. If it has been 5 years since it was out in public last, then maybe there is a reason for that.

"Do I want to wear you again?"

Maybe you have replaced it with a new and nicer version, but since you two have had so many good experiences together, you have kept it. It is all about respecting the story, but still...

"Do I simply use you or are you simply usable?"

Perhaps it is time to say goodbye and thanks. You have had a long life together, but have grown apart. Maybe it's the size, maybe the fashion—you have no future together anymore.

"What value do you bring to me?"

Maybe the dress is both nice, new, expensive and neat, but if you just do not feel that you get your value's worth wearing it, then you must go your separate ways.

"Do I want to spend the time and money in repair?"

It does not take much damage before one piece of clothing gets left in the closet. Maybe the zipper in your favourite jeans broke and they will never be the same again.

"How long have you been hanging there for?"

You may be surprised how old some of your clothes really are. Clothing with TOO many chances.

"How many do I need?"

Here, you might get rid of clothing that may even be new, but you simply have too much—or too many. How many jeans do you need? How many T-shirts? How many black ankle socks? Select the best ones and keep them.

"How many dress-up clothes should I save for the grandchildren?"

Most of us probably loved diving into our grandmother's wardrobe as a child and dressing up as an elegant lady. But that does not justify your mess. Nobody says that your wardrobe should be an authentic theatre wardrobe for your grandchildren to come and dress up maybe once every two years. Maybe you need one of the boxes for this. Maybe!

This is how you do it

Take one shelf at a time and think only in two categories to begin with:

Wearing/not wearing

When you take only one shelf at a time, you can manage the process. Maybe the clothing has to be reorganized afterwards, but we will deal with that when the time is right.

You have to be completely honest

Take out a pile of blouses. Take one blouse at a time. When you start talking to your clothes, you should immediately decide where it should go. You already know whether or not you are using it. Forget about your bad conscience. Also, do not fool yourself into thinking that you might wear that blouse when you actually forgot you had it. That is just another bad excuse. If you have not worn it, there is a reason for it.

Right now, it is about cleaning up and clearing out the closet. Make a quick decision. Remember, it is about 'wearing' or 'not wearing'.

NOTE! Use the opportunity to be a bit critical. Maybe that T-shirt needs to be replaced.

Remember it is about the
highest common denominator
– you deserve the best!

Clothing you are 100% certain that you wear, fold nicely and put it back on the shelf.

Managing clothing you do not wear
Hopefully you now have a huge pile of clothing that did not make the cut.

Again, there are only 2 categories for this pile of clothing:

1. Recycling
2. Throwing out

We need to make sure that clothing in the recycling category is clean and without damages. The recipient should not need to repair it—no matter who it is. There is probably a reason why you have not repaired it after all this time…

Recycling

Clothing suitable for recycling is:

- Clothing to a second-hand store
- Clothing to friends or family
- Clothing to be re-sold

Now fold everything nicely that needs to be recycled and put it in bags clearly marked where it is going to. 'Recycling', 'sister', 'online sale'...

Remember, it is forbidden to export your mess to others. If you want to pass things on to friends and family, you have to have their true consent!

Exporting clutter is strictly forbidden!

Section Out

Clothing in this pile should not be paid too much attention. Simply OUT. You can throw it in a clothing container where it will be recycled—regardless of its condition, since the non-wearable will be ripped apart and reused in a different version.

Down to the detail

So far, we have only talked about clothing as a general term. Now we are truly going into details, focusing on each individual piece, whether it is clothing or things.

Underwear

Go through all your underwear and save only the best. Forget about bras with too many years on the straps. It is fine with all the sets of underwear, but panties are being washed more often than bras. Are there too many bras in fun colours laying around without panties?

Socks

Black ankle socks do not cost a fortune. Throw out all the pairs that no longer look nice.

How do your nylons look? The half ones and the long ones. Do they still have a match?

Tights? And the thicker ones? Are they worn on the foot? Discoloured?

Cardigans, sweaters, pullovers

They do not last forever. Keep only the very best of the ones you are using. The ones not worn down by washing and those with all the buttons intact.

Shirts, tunics

How many do you need? Keep only the best ones. Imagine leaving for two weeks and having to pick six. Which ones would you grab?

Seasonal clothing

Not all clothing is being used year-round. Some clothing is being used quite well, whether it is summer or winter. Only the accessories change. But we also have clothing that is strictly seasonal.

Make a box for storing seasonal clothing. If you have a solid rack in the basement, use moving boxes. A big plastic storage box will also do. You just have to be able to write on it that it is seasonal clothing.

When it is time, either one way or another, the content is to be changed. Before throwing things in the box, remember to ask the dress if you want to see it again next season.

Skiwear

Skiwear is of course also part of seasonal clothing. Create a box especially for all clothing that belongs here. Remember to get rid of skiwear you do not use anymore. As it is rarely worn down, recycle it.

A small tip

Ski jackets and pants have a tendency to take up a lot of room. Roll them firmly and then put them in a freezer bag of an appropriate size. A 2 or 4 litre bag is usually adequate. Shape it a bit, it pays off. You can almost reduce a ski jacket to a fifth of its size. Also use this tip when packing for your ski holiday.

Sportswear

Maybe you used to be a cycling enthusiast a couple of years ago, but then the interest died. I know that all the gear including clothing costs a bundle, but there is a reason why you quit the passion.

Work clothes

Now you are probably thinking that you would also like to look decent when doing yard work or painting. Of course. But it also has its limit. Even clothes for painting can go out-of-fashion. Sure, you may still be able to fit the jeans you used for painting 10 years ago, but even this type of clothing is allowed to evolve a bit when it comes to fashion, after all. And how much of it do you need?

Jackets

How about jackets? Jackets are not worn a lot, and it might be a bit difficult saying goodbye to them. They are usually expensive. But the jacket will be neither more beautiful nor more modern because of this. Recycle them.

The revealing trick

Once you have been through all the glory, use this small trick and flip all the hangers, so the hook faces the wrong way. As you wear it, place the hanger the right way around.

Once six months have passed, you can clearly see what you have and have not used, and therefore what needs to be thrown out.

Hangers – by the way

Now that we are talking about hangers, take a look at the hangers in your wardrobe. In my time, I have seen wardrobes with far more than 50 different hangers on the bar. Frankly—it's not a pretty sight.

Hangers do not cost a fortune and you will feel at ease and satisfied when looking at a bar with identical hangers. Buy plenty and buy hangers with 'round shoulders'. They do not have to be suit hangers, just simple plastic hangers with rounded ends so you avoid pointy shoulders in your jackets. This can quickly move a jacket to the 'not-wearing pile'.

Folding technique

What good does it do reducing your wardrobe from 100 to 20%, if everything is just lying around on the shelves?

Clothing needs to be folded neatly

Use a table when you fold clothes after washing. Clothing that is air-folded will never be sharp at the edges and will therefore appear used before you wear it. This does not increase the usefulness.

Clean clothes are folded in lines and put nicely on the shelf. Socks are paired and put together neatly. It will save you a lot of time when you are looking for 2 identical ones in the morning.

Button the top button on your shirts when hanging on the hanger - it makes the collar a lot nicer.

Worn but not dirty clothing

Clothes can easily be used several times. Because you have worn a blouse a couple of hours does not mean it has to be washed. With a bit of sensible recycling you protect, not only your clothes, but also your wallet and the environment.

Nevertheless, it is nice to know the difference between clean and slightly worn clothes. A blouse that has only been worn a little and can be used again, should be folded in the middle the long way. Not like a clean one, where the sleeves are folded towards the centre. By using another folding technique for clothing, you have worn just a little, you can always see if it is a completely clean or less clean blouse on the shelf.

Shoes

It had to come... How does the shoe section look?

Here you must be very, very critical. Shoes that have been worn throughout the years are wonderful to wear; but how pretty are they?

Shoes have a tendency to hang around longer than they should. You know which ones you want to wear. All shoes are not favourite shoes, and even if they are your favourite sandals, they might not be as pretty as they used to be.

Here, you really have to stay sharp when asking. Talk to your shoes and keep only the best ones. Also remember seasonal storage here. Remove winter boots until next season.

Jewellery

Jewellery is also not modern forever. Sorry.

Things carried very close to the body are more difficult to get rid of—especially jewellery. It almost does not matter whether it is expensive or cheap jewellery. They simply cling on and they are not worn down.

If you have valuable pieces of jewellery that you do not use anymore, consider selling them. If you are lucky enough that they are made of gold, there might even be a decent financial gain if you sell them by weight.

Choose to recycle the less valuable jewellery. Even mediocre plastic jewellery can be valuable for someone who is attending an 80's party and is looking for accessories in a second-hand store.

Scarves

It is a bit the same with scarves. It is not easy to say goodbye to these and they are not worn down either. But that does not imply that we should keep them forever—or until a moth family comes over and makes the decision for us.

Because it has been decorative once does not imply that it still is. Allow yourself a bit of renewal.

Bags

Bags are usually also made of a reasonably solid material. At least those we have not already thrown out.

Keep only those you have used in the last year. You will probably not use the rest. Send them off to recycling if it is still in good shape.

Organizing and Storage

It is now time to look at some good solutions on how to store things in your wardrobe. Of course, there are many solutions from simple shelves to a top-of-the-line designed closet, where nothing is left to chance.

As most of us do, you probably have an ordinary closet and you should not be unhappy about that. Just make the most of it. You can pick from the following outlined solutions and use what feels best for you.

Closet and shelves

Now organize your clothes so that pants hang together, shirts hang together, dresses hang together, etc.

Also organize the shelves so that tops without sleeves are in the same pile, T-shirts in the same pile and long-sleeved blouses in the same pile. Now put it all in proper stacks.

It does not hurt that it also looks nice when you look at the newly created order and finding the right thing will be much easier.

Shoes

There is a multitude of different solutions for storing shoes. Most require a certain amount of patience to use, which is far from present in most shoe users. But if you can manage to put your shoes in pockets every time you take them off, then that it is a suitable solution for you.

If you are one of those kicking off your shoes into the bottom of the wardrobe, then put a small shelf, 7cm in height is enough, at floor height, so shoes do not fall onto the floor or get stuck in the sliding door. Or put a large, but low box in the bottom of your closet. If you have a suitable wall, put up some long shelves at foot height.

If you have an outside closet gable or a suitable wall, you can put up an IKEA Bygel bar and hang your lovely high-heeled shoes by their heel for decoration.

Party shoes are of course stored in nice boxes. Maybe even with a window.

IKEA also has excellent narrow boxes for hanging on the wall for shoe storage. They do not fit in a wardrobe, but they hang nicely in an entrance hall for example. It is often here that shoes are thrown on and off, so maybe it is time to move shoes out of the wardrobe. It will also improve the indoor aroma in the wardrobe...

If you have space for a closet with a depth of only 30cm, you can put up shelves closely together and make room for plenty of shoes. Buy one 60cm in width and possibly put it with its backside against your closet gable. Or if you have an unused corner between two closets, fill it with shelves for shoes.

Buy a Scholl Shoe Fresh to improve the quality of the aroma in your trainers—and in the closet.

Underwear and socks

Make it easy for yourself. Many wardrobe manufacturers make drawers with compartments. Nice compartments, where there is room for a nice set of underwear or similar. I think this is an excellent solution—IF ONLY YOU HAVE PATIENCE TO USE IT. Otherwise, it is not practical at all.

If it fits into your closet solution, get some plastic baskets of some kind that you like and put panties in one, bras in another and socks in a third and fourth. This makes it much easier for you to clean up and put in place.

Be careful not to over-organize.
Life should be easy.

Ties and belts

Here we get into the men's department a bit, but a little order in your partner's things is also appropriate.

The previously mentioned space dividers are amazing for ties and belts. There are many nice tie hangers and it is excellent if you have the patience. Otherwise, it is quick to roll up a tie and put it in the drawer.

Belts, we are on common ground again. Belts can also be placed perfectly in these compartments. IKEA even has some nice white boxes which fit into most drawers.

Or hang the belt on a hanger by pulling the belt buckle over the hook. If you can put up a rack, this is also good for belts.

Jewellery

There are lots of things for hanging bracelets and necklaces. An alternative could once again be a Bygel from IKEA for you to hang them.

A 'jewellery dress' seen at containerstore.com or a good old-fashioned sock organizer with lots of pockets hanging on a hanger is also an excellent solution for storing jewellery in the closet, as it does not take up a lot of room, but has a lot of space inside.

I have also seen a mirror with a hidden space behind the mirror. You just open the mirror as a door and behind this you find hidden space with a lot of hooks.

Ear studs and rings

For small things like ear studs and rings, I can recommend chocolate boxes. Yes, you read correctly. Those boxes that are divided into small tiny compartments. If you are lucky enough to receive a box of delicious chocolates, it is often in a box where there is even clear plastic in the lid. Otherwise, just use the box without a lid.

Bags you use every day

We will once again need a wall of a suitable size and a bar. For example, Bygel from IKEA.

Furthermore, you will need a number of hooks. Again IKEA—or another manufacturer. Put up the hook and hang the bag. Put small bags in a suitable spacious basket.

Tips for storing bags

Bags are best to be stored in bags. Pack them inside each other or put them in the big bag basket you bought on your last trip to France or in your weekend suitcase.

The Full Overview

By now you should have reduced the inside of your wardrobe so what you see is only the best of the best. Clothes that represent you. Clothing that tells the right story about who you are.

You will have such a good overview of your clothing that you can also see if something is missing.

Should there be a couple of holes, you can afford to fill them now that you have taken full control over your wardrobe. No more excess or mistaken purchases anymore.

Ugh, why did I throw that out?

Yes, at some point you will think to yourself how in the world could you throw out that hot little skirt?

Listen carefully: This happened because you do not have it in front of you and remember it as it looked in its glory days—and not as it looked after you wore it for 5 years, washing it over and over again—and last time not without incident.

We forget the facts. We forget that our clothes got older when we do not have them in front of us anymore. I also prefer not looking at myself too much in the mirror to be reminded that days go by. But that does not change the facts...

Therefore, yes, at some point you will feel regret, but trust yourself that you made the right decision when you said goodbye to the worn camel wool sweater after a long and faithful companionship.

The Permanent Order

So far so good, but do not think that everything is done just because you have sorted out your belongings. Removing clutter and maintaining order are two different things. Now you must embrace new habits in your life. Otherwise all the trouble will go to waste. That would be a shame.

"Clutter is like a weed. You have to keep it down or it will take control."

Clearly, there are some routines in your daily life that you will have to change. The good news is that it does not hurt and it is not as difficult as you might think. Your job is simply to change your way of thinking a little.

How to keep only treasures in your wardrobe

So far so good, but do not think that your wardrobe would like to be a treasure chest filled with your treasures for the rest of your life, as you continue to buy stuff that does not correspond with you.

From now on, every time you buy a new piece of clothing you must talk with it before you swipe your credit card.

The key question is: Are we going to best friends forever?

If the answer is not a loud YES, you are not made for each other. Say goodbye and leave it.

How to keep order in your wardrobe

Order in your wardrobe does not come naturally. You must care for it and keep a close eye on it. Do not ever become lazy by not caring.

Every piece of clothing in your wardrobe is a piece of you, and no one in the world deserves more care than you. Every time you touch a piece of clothing, you touch yourself. Promise me to care.

Whenever you bring your clothing back from being washed or simply replace something slightly used, you must care for it and fold it properly. If you just throw it onto a random shelf you will never grab it as your first choice next time.

How to keep order anywhere forever

The best way to keep order in your wardrobe, or anywhere else, is to close circles behind you.

The secret is to keep active clutter from becoming passive clutter. Once you have finished something, it must be cleaned up, even on a small scale.

Imagine that every task that you perform runs in circles. You start one place and end in the same place. Each time you finish one round, everything should be back in place, ready for another round. Some circles overlap, but they still have their own course. All circles are chores, tasks or projects in a closed circle. They always have a start and an end. Once the chore is finished, it has reached its expiration.

This way, you can greatly reduce the amount of time that you spend cleaning up after yourself. You can invest your time better because you do not return to the clutter two or ten times before you are finished cleaning up. You just need to continuously maintain your trail in order once you finish a chore or task.

If you do not clean up afterwards, the task will hang in the air until it is finished.

How to maintain the treasures

You must be the guardian of the standard of the clothes in your wardrobe. Everything has to be in perfect order. If a button becomes lose, sew it on immediately, otherwise you have just moved your favourite cardigan closer to the waste basket.

Take care of your shoes and protect them against rain and dirt. Your shoes will love you for it.

How to watch for expiration dates

Everything has an expiration date. I truly mean EVERYTHING.

We have a lifelong partnership with some things and the expiration date with these will be the same as our own, but the vast majority of your clutter has probably exceeded its limit. If you do not use something, it is meaningless to you. It has reached the end. You have used up that specific piece. You do not have a common path anymore and it is time to separate.

If you do not get rid of whatever it is, it will start to drain you of energy. You will get annoyed with it and feel guilty for not having made the decision to throw it out. The thing owns you now, instead of vice versa. It has become a parasite.

When you and your jeans do not fit each other anymore, they have reached the expiration date. You must get rid of them at once. Out.

Bonus Section - Duvets

Funnily enough, there are often extra duvets in the closet. Do you have duvets in your wardrobe? And if your guest duvet is one of your own old duvets, throw it out. Dust mites live off our dead skin. They only die at high temperature, which is not the case when dry cleaning. Even if you wash the duvet, the result is only freshly washed dust mites, as they are still living in the duvet. Arghh. Allow yourself a fresh duvet once in a while.

If you have extra duvets lying on the top section of the closet, then buy a cheap plastic handbag with hooks and a zipper. But buy only the little ones, approx. 30x10x40cm. It is large enough for a duvet when it is rolled and compressed well before it is put in the bag. The advantage of this bag is that the duvet does not expand more than the bag allows. I know the trick with the black bag and vacuum cleaner, but it does not last. A small tiny hole in the bag and the duvet fills up the bag. Furthermore, the shape is not very practical.

Bed linen

Are you also the kind of person that cannot go to IKEA without returning with new bed linen?

And here we have the problem: Bed linen are not worn down, which means it is too good to throw out...

True, but how many sets do you need? How often do you have hordes of overnight guests who do not know that one brings their own bed linen? Never, right?

How to get smooth bed linen

If you tumble dry your bed linen, take it out while it is still a little damp. Fold it half way, nicely. Hang it over the clothesline and smooth it with your hand. When dry, fold it completely. Again nicely. It is so nice having a clean bed with nice bed linen after just a bit of extra care.

If you dry your bed linen outside in the fresh air, great, let it dry when the weather is nice and windy. And then fold it neatly.

To Sum Up

- Talk to your things.
- There is so much you can use, but so little you need.
- Remember, it is about minimizing— otherwise you are right back where you started.
- Do not settle—then better to do without.
- Keep only the best.
- Things and clothing do not become more modern by keeping them.
- Do not export your clutter to others.
- Fold clothing neatly.
- How many do you need of one kind?
- Who are you keeping it for? Yourself or others?
- Use seasonal storage.
- Close circles behind you to avoid clutter from piling up.

At the End

By now, you should know a lot of good tips on how to get started on organizing your wardrobe so you can quickly find the 20% of gold that is no longer hiding.

Enjoy knowing what you have in your wardrobe so that you can decide in a split-second whether or not you need that lovely thing when temptation arises in some store. What does it go with? Do I need it? And buy something really nice when you know it is exactly what you want.

You deserve the best!

Afterword

Dear reader, that is all I want to teach you for now. I hope that you will enjoy and use every bit of information I have given you, and that it will bring you the order that you have been looking for.

Sign up for my newsletter and we will stay in touch: lenabentsen.com

If you have enjoyed the book, I will be very happy if you would review it on Amazon.

If you have comments, please feel free to contact me here: contact@lenabentsen.com

Other Books by Lena Bentsen

<u>Available on Amazon:</u>

- Goodbye Clutter, Hello Freedom: How to create space for Danish Hygge and Lifestyle by decluttering, organizing and decorating with care

<u>Coming soon in English:</u>

- The Secret to Danish Hygge: How to create, live and enjoy the Danish lifestyle
- Enjoy Your Move: The Danish hygge and decluttering guide to downsize and style your house for sale, pack and move, and settle in to your new home with joy
- Enjoy Your Christmas Time: How to create the perfect December with Danish Hygge and no stress
- Enjoy Your Kitchen: How to revamp, optimize and organize in 5 easy steps
- Enjoy Your Work Desk: How to regain control by decluttering and organizing
- Enjoy Your Everyday Life: How to get off the hamster wheel with 5 magic circles
- Enjoy Love and Life: 11 ways to boost your self-worth and become the best YOU

Learn more at lenabentsen.com
or Facebook @danishhygge

Made in the USA
Columbia, SC
19 September 2018